Behcet's, Sutton's, Lyme Disease or Candida? The Non-Sexually Acquired Rash That Just Won't Go Away

Organic Living Publishing
All rights reserved
ISBN: 9781092755306

Table Of Contents

1. How It All Begins — 4
2. The Importance of Getting Properly Diagnosed — 6
3. What is Behcet's Syndrome? — 11
4. How Do We know It's Not Sutton's Disease, Also Known as NSAGU or NAGU (Nonsexually Aquired Genital Ulceration)? — 14
5. Stress as a Contributing Factor — 17
6. Is It Lyme Disease? — 20
7. What is Lyme Disease? — 22
8. Potentiation — 24
9. Harmful Microorganisms — 26
10. Electromagnetic Radiation (EMR) — 33
11. Autoimmunity — 35
12. Zinc Oxide -- Cheap and Effective — 39
13. Detoxing the Kidneys and the Bladder — 41
14. Detox Protocol — 43
15. References — 49

How It All Begins

There are many things that happen in the lives of women that can cause trauma, heartache or pain. The frustration of struggling with a rash that just won't go away ranks high on the scale of gut wrenching experiences.

Dumbfounded by the amount of calls I get from women tearfully describing chronic what they think are yeast infections, I have gone on a quest of searching for a cause. What I have uncovered is vast, theoretically sound and unfortunately, little known as of yet. One of the primary obstacles is proper diagnosis.

The saga often starts with herpetic, yeast or bacterial vaginosis diagnoses, except that then it just lingers, and lingers, and lingers....sometimes for years. Eventually, women just give up. They just focus on keeping the area clean, baths, creams...and sometimes even antidepressants. Many resign going to doctors, while others see a specialist after a specialist to get non-specific inflammatory dermatitis definitions, atrophic vaginitis, chronic bacterial vaginosis or worse yet, wrong fungal diagnoses to be addressed with futile fungicides.

What makes things even worse, is the sensitive nature of it all. How do we even talk about it?

The Importance of Getting Properly Diagnosed

A number of women faced with what they perceive as chronic candida won't see a doctor at all. And that number, based on internet forums, is alarmingly large.

Behcet's, Sutton, candida...? What is it? What if it's a diagnosis that simply cannot be faced right now?

Behcet's Disease, or Syndrome, (which turns out may be the diagnosis for many) is currently classified as a rare disease because fewer than 20,000 new cases are logged in each year in the United States. Many men and women suffering today, may have viral, fungal or bacterial infections, for which we have more than adequate medications. There is no reason for them to suffer needlessly.

For what I believe is the majority, however, we are looking at a heavy metal toxicity. With a proper detox, these patients start improving within 48 hours. What's even more exciting is that the course of treatment is simple, non-toxic, inexpensive and effective. First, we have to make sure that we are dealing with the right demon.

Is it herpetic? For those of us who have had mouth cold sores, the signs of herpes are unmistakable -- small, liquid-filled blisters that burn with a prickly sensation, then burst, crust and heal. The entire ordeal is normally resolved within 2-3 weeks, although in some instances, the sores may take up several months to heal. Herpes is often the first diagnosis people with genital outbreaks get, mostly because of its prevalence. Sadly, testing for herpes produces a slew of false positives, with 1 in 2 tests turning up false positive results.

And what happens when the sores don't go away?

Is it candida? Candidiasis is also easy to diagnose and just as easy to recognize due to the white cottage cheese-like discharge and persistent itch. Unfortunately, it's a common co-infection, so for many women, that is where the struggle begins. And again, it just doesn't go away.

Commonly, women's initial discomfort is initiated right *after* taking antibiotics. Others feel that their antifungal medications prompt or exacerbate their chronic conditions. The link may or may not be clearly established, but the correlation is there.

Since correlation does not equal causation, there are some important questions we need to ask. Why were you prescribed an antibiotic? Did you find a tick on your body and take Doxycycline preventatively? Do you have a history of allergies or skin conditions? And of course, did you see a dermatologist, not just your GYN?

I am finding it more and more common for women to have had a tick bite, or to have engaged in physical activities in nature, prior to onset. Wondering about a possible Lyme Disease connection, I turned to colleagues to inquire about their experiences. Naturopaths immediately point to heavy metal toxins. I was seeking a Lyme Disease connection, so I asked an MD friend of mine if she has been acquainted with the types of situations where Lyme Disease infections cause genital ulcers and rashes. She said, no, but she said, "It's possibly autoimmune. Like the aphthous ulcers people get in their mouths."

I believe it is important to note that the specific patient I was inquiring about has seen a number of doctors and has gotten no real diagnosis. Her condition has persisted for years. She is in her 40s.

That makes the situation even more dire. Now what? As a society, we have resigned ourselves to the idea that autoimmune conditions are prompted by our confused bodies that attack themselves for no reason, and there is nothing that can be done. We are told there is no cure, just maintenance.

What is this aphthous ulcer autoimmune condition?

What is Behcet's Syndrome?

According to the American Behcet's Disease association, "Behcet's Disease, also known as Behcet's syndrome, is a rare, chronic, autoimmune, autoinflammatory disorder of unknown origin. Its manifestations are thought to be caused by vasculitis resulting in damage to blood vessels throughout the body. The disease is named for the Turkish dermatologist, Dr. Hulusi Behcet, who in 1937, described a triad of oral ulcers, genital ulcers and ocular inflammation. Although Behcet's Disease is recognized worldwide, prevalence is highest in countries in the eastern Mediterranean...Behcet's Disease tends to develop in young adults, typically in their 20's and 30's, but patients of all ages, gender and races may be affected." [1]

Confusion ensues as people tend to think that their mouths and eyes also need to be affected. Behçet's Disease may occur at different sites -- skin, eyes, heart, kidneys, gastrointestinal tract, joints, blood vessels, etc. Like with all autoimmune conditions, treatment options focus on management of symptoms.

To make matters worse, many people suffering are now are older and report a change in the type of rash over time. Sometimes deep classic aphthous ulcers morph into skin lesions around the labia, on the outside of the vagina, as an itch on the anus or on the crease by the thighs. Sometimes it's just an itchy rash. If the patient is in menopause, atrophic vaginitis is often considered. Lab tests that point to autoimmunity and/or to rule out cancerous conditions follow.

Trichomoniasis, a parasite that's normally, but not always, spread through sex, must also be ruled out. Scabies must also be considered. These tiny human mites burrow into our skin causing severe itchiness, especially at night.

On their quest for answers, my patients often consider contact dermatitis caused by soaps, perfumes, dyes, non-organic cotton, pads, tampons, laundry detergents, fabrics and more. Psoriasis is also not ruled out, especially in those prone to skin conditions.

How Do We know It's Not Sutton's Disease, Also Known as NSAGU or NAGU (Nonsexually Aquired Genital Ulceration)?

Behcet's or Sutton's? The difference is difficult to establish, as Sutton's is a little understood condition that causes canker sore-like ulcers in the mouth and on the genitals as well. Is it possible that Behcet's and Sutton's have merged today to form a different type of non-sexually acquired genital ulcers potentiated by our ever-changing environment? Stress, a compromised immune system, injury or deficiencies in iron, vitamin B12, and folate may also play a role.

Unlike the canker sore, commonly caused by the herpes virus, this type of an ulcer is a non-sexually acquired autoimmune response to the bacteria normally present in mucus membranes. It is considered benign and its onset may be triggered by a viral infection. Sutton's is also known as NSAGU, NAGU, Lipshutz ulcer, vulvar aphthae and complex aphthosis.[3] This terminology confuses women even more.

One group of Australian physicians, says it best, "Aphthous ulceration is a harmless condition. A tendency to aphthae runs in families. The cause is still unknown...Attacks of aphthous ulcers are often recurrent ranging from infrequent to very frequent, to the point where they are almost constant."

This group is called A Care Down There and it comprises dermatologists, gynaecologists, a pain management specialist, a sexual health physician, a psychologist, and a pelvic floor physiotherapist. Their advice? See your doctor and get a prescription for Doxycycline to prevent recurrence. They ask that you direct your GP to their website, as many general practitioners are not adept at dealing with recurrent genital ulcers.[4]

Stress as a Contributing Factor

We live in a world marred with pollution. Driving long hours to get to thankless, stress-filled cubicles -- where we address passive aggressive co-workers, reporting to disconnected management, under constant fire for performance -- has become the norm.

The human bot wasn't designed to function this way. Our bodies have been programmed to alternate between sympathetic and parasympathetic responses. The sympathetic response, our normal on the go fight-or-flight mechanism, must be counterbalanced by the rest-and-digest system -- the mode, under which self-healing and repair take place. Unfortunately, for most of us, this mode is under a continual barrage of daily stressors, a mode robbed of respite, calm and all things essential to our very survival. My book, Stress,

Inflammation, and Quantum Possibilities, shares extensive research into the American way of life and our unhealthy relationship with rest and relaxation.

Parasympathetic, also known as rest-and-restore responses are vital. It is of no surprise then, that patients with autoimmune conditions often describe stress as a precursor to their condition, only to be augmented by the discomfort that follows.

There are many, many ways in which stress can be addressed. Some people like hiking, exercising, singing or painting, while others prefer regular massages, self-care and biofeedback. Whatever your drug of choice, please make a note-to-self and follow through no matter how meaningless or needless self-care may appear at the time, especially when you feel too stressed to be able to relax altogether. That is actually, when you need it most.

Biofeedback is becoming one of the fastest growing lifestyle intervention therapies for managing stress. Combined with aromatherapy, acupuncture, Qigong, yoga and regular massages, it has the potential to change lives and the outcomes of conditions previously deemed untreatable.

We know that chronic stress is at the root of all autoimmune conditions. That is why parasympathetic/relaxation response treatments are absolutely essential to any therapeutic regimen.

Is It Lyme Disease?

A genital rash, as a symptom of Lyme Disease, may seem absurd, but research confirms that this type of manifestation may not be as far-fetched as it appears to be at a first glance.

According to an article published in JAMA, a 50 year old with Sutton's (NAGU) resolved her symptoms after being treated for Lyme Disease with 100mg of Doxycycline twice daily. Is it a coincidence that the Australian team suggested the same type of a treatment?

JAMA also suggests an infectious etiology in these types of cases, but in more than 75% of patients, pathogens are never identified. In the other 25%, Mycoplasma, the Epstein-Barr Virus, aerobic bacteria, HIV, mumps, cytomegalovirus, influenza A, and *Toxoplasma gondii* and now LYME disease have been associated with Sutton's (NAGU).

"...we can consider NAGU among the protean immunologic manifestations of Lyme disease. Lyme titer analysis should be considered for women presenting with genital ulcers of unclear etiology." (JAMA, 2014)[5]

What Is Lyme Disease?

Lyme disease is a tick-borne affliction caused by Borrelia burgdorferi -- a bacterium that *initially causes* headaches, fever, fatigue, and a characteristic skin rash called erythema migrans. Untreated, the infection can spread to the joints, the brain, the heart, and the entire nervous system.

Current diagnosis of Lyme disease is based on symptoms and laboratory tests called ELISA and Western Blot. Although, ELISA is tested first and then confirmed by Western Blot, some practitioners prefer to run both tests, as ELISA has been found to be largely inaccurate, especially if the infection is less than a month old.

Although Lyme disease can be treated effectively with a several week-long course of antibiotics, new research suggests that the standard 28-day treatments may not be sufficient. Moreover, Lyme Disease can transmit other tick-borne diseases such as anaplasmosis, mycoplasmosis, babesiosis, bartonellosis, ehrlichiosis, Rocky Mountain spotted fever, and more.[6]

Potentiation

Potentiation refers to the influences that enable the spread of a disease, therefore factors that potentiate a condition, envelope causes that strengthen its virulence.

Causes that potentiate Lyme Disease chronic manifestations (outside of stress and a compromised immune system) are not widely accepted.

In spite of criticism, one man stands out from the crowd. That man is Dr. Dietrich Klinghardt, MD and PhD known for his successful integrative treatments of neurological disorders, Lyme Disease, and chronic pain.

Because today's definition of Lyme Disease refers to *illnesses transferred by insects, mosquitoes, spiders, fleas and mites* (not just ticks), the top naturopathic Lyme Disease physician -- who is also a PhD and an MD -- Dr. Dietrich Klinghardt, believes infections are more common than previously suspected.

Not only are they more common, they are more virulent too. What potentiates them?

"I personally suspect that the exposure to electromagnetic fields in the home and the microwaves from cell phone radiation are driving the virulence of many of the microbes that are naturally in us, and makes them aggressive and illness producing." ~ Dr. Dietrich Klinghardt, MD, PhD[7]

Harmful Microorganisms

The WHO (The World Health Organization) has a division called the International Agency for the Research of Cancer. It evaluates electromagnetic fields (EMFs), and it is vetted for conflicts of interest. The organization is considered to be the gold standard for evaluating carcinogens.

The International Agency for Research on Cancer classifies radio frequencies as a Class 2B carcinogen. These frequencies include sources such as cell phones, laptops, tablets, baby monitors, WiFi, cell towers...anything in the range of 30KHz to 300GHz. Many independently working scientists and members of the academia agree. They posit that the scientific evidence is substantial enough to conclude that radiofrequency radiation is a human carcinogen.

Electromagnetic smog also has an effect on our biology, on parasites, molds and mycotoxins. Examples of harmful mycotoxins include aflatoxin, fumonisins, ochratoxin A, patulin, citrinin, trichothecenes, zearalenone, and more. In addition, one mold species may produce many different mycotoxins, and several species may produce the same mycotoxin.

These mycotoxins, potentiated by electromagnetic radiation (EMR) can make us sick, producing symptoms such as:

- Chronic sore throat
- Recurrent rashes, especially where bodily fluids are present
- Systemic inflammation
- Digestive irregularities (bloating, constipation or diarrhea)
- Burning or clogged nasal passages

- Brain fog, dizziness or tremors
- Breathing problems
- Loss of balance
- Constant low grade depression (loss of zest for life)
- Anxiety or insomnia
- Eye irritation
- Chronic fatigue
- Headaches
- Chronic yeast infections, and more

How do we know that potentiation from EMR takes place?

The answer comes from a Swiss physician, who grew mold cultures under a Faraday cage -- a silver canape of fine netting. He meticulously measured the amount of toxins these molds were producing on a daily basis. During the second part of the experiment, he exposed the culture to the normal electromagnetic radiation in his laboratory, which was influenced by a cell phone, a laptop, lights and the cell tower that was nearby. Amazingly, the production of mycotoxins went up over than 600 times, as the mold produced a huge number of mycotoxins to protect itself. In addition, these strains were a lot more viscous and virulent.[9]

The connection between mycotoxins and Chronic Fatigue Syndrome (CFS) is also well documented. Scientific studies have recognized mold as a serious health risk by conducting research at water-damaged buildings.

Patients with CFS were evaluated for mold exposure and their urine was tested for mycotoxins using Enzyme Linked

Immunosorbent Assays (ELISA) -- the same test we use when diagnosing Lyme Disease. 93% of the people studied were positive for at least one mycotoxin.

Another sample of healthy adults, with no history of chronic exposure to mold, revealed no positive cases. It is important to note that the testing was done by the same lab, using the same research methodology.[10]

Since 75% to 80% of our immune responses are linked to gut heath, we must ask ourselves if mycotoxins affect gut flora and microbiota as well.

Researchers at the Department of Nutrition and Dietetics at the Faculty of Medicine and Health Sciences at the Universiti Putra, Malaysia, have found a connection. They concluded that metabolites produced by mycotoxins, are capable of causing diseases and death in humans and animals. Mycotoxins caused gut issues, particularly in the epithelial tissues.

The gut microbiota should be capable of eliminating mycotoxins, unless the beneficial bacteria have been compromised by pathogens. Given the outcome, the study concluded that prevention and therapy of mycotoxin contamination is of utmost importance.[11]

Mold toxin illness is also a reason why some individuals with Lyme disease have difficulty recovering.

Dr. Marty Ross, MD writes that lowering inflammatory cytokines is essential for Lyme disease recovery. Cytokines are proteins made by the white blood cells to help our immune system. In excess, they may cause Lyme disease symptoms.[12]

Mold Toxin Illness is a complex matter. Dr. Joseph Brewer, M.D. is an infectious disease specialist, who theorizes that an ongoing source for mold toxins is colonization of the sinus passages in the adults he studied. His presentation to the 2013 International Lyme and Associated Diseases annual scientific conference included unpublished findings supporting the benefits of treating mold with nasal irrigation using antifungal and fat binding medications such as cholestyramine. He noted that the treatment path lasts for months and is linked to mold mitigation.[13]

Now that we know that mold potentiates Lyme and EMR potentiates mold, a primary course of treatment should involve cleaning up the electromagnetic smog in our environment.

Electromagnetic Radiation (EMR)

How do we clear the electromagnetic radiation (EMR) from our environment?

Start with a safe sleeping space. Ideally, this would be a room with no TV, no electric appliances, cell phones or computers. It would be painted with shungite paint, have EMF protective film on the windows, and all electricity should be turned off in the entire house right from the control panel. There would be no wireless phones in the house, no smart meter, and the bed will be enveloped with a Faraday cage in the form of a silver threaded canape.

It is important to note that there should be zero cell phone or wireless computer use taking place in this room. Stetzer filters should don each outlet.

If you are sick, consider EMF protected (silver threaded) underwear, grounded pillow cases, grounding mats that emit negative ions, and more.

Autoimmunity

Do you ever stop and think why every second person you know is battling an autoimmune condition? What do you think it is causing such confusion that the body starts attacking itself, as the definition of an autoimmune condition suggests? How many people around you have Hashimoto's, Crohn's Disease, Fibromyalgia or Rheumatoid Arthritis (RA)? Is their condition related to an underlying chronic infection? Which one?

It has been long speculated that Hashimoto's is linked to re-animation of the Epstein Barr Virus (EBV), the same virus from the herpes family that in some cases causes mono. It is estimated that 95% of the population carries it, although many have never exhibited symptoms. The EBV virus, HSV4, lays dormant in most Americans. A study conducted by the

Department of Histology and Embryology, and the Department of Physiotherapy at the Medical University of Silesia in Poland concluded that "EBV is not the only agent responsible for the development of autoimmune thyroid diseases. However, it can be considered a contributory factor."[14]

Fibromyalgia may be also linked to a herpes virus. HSV6, to be precise. Roseola. Roseola is what most kids today get instead of the chicken pox, since most are vaccinated. Roseola is a mutation of the chicken pox virus, another virus from the herpes family. The Nuffield Department of Clinical Neurosciences at the University of Oxford in the United Kingdom, has published a study concluding that herpes simplex virus type 1 (HSV1) is a major risk for Alzheimer's disease (AD). That study cites 72 additional references.[15]

Could an autoimmune aphthous ulcer be reanimated HSV virus of some sort? Even HSV2, but chronic, due to a compromised immune system? Most patients turn up positive for HSV1 and 2, as that test only points to an exposure and most of us have it. That exposure does not have to be sexually acquired, and I believe that often it is not. One of the primary reasons, for which we disqualify HSV1 or HSV2 as condentors, are the chronic characteristics and the autoimmune nature of this never-ending skin condition.

Yet consider herpes zoster (shingles). As a reanimated chicken pox herpetic infection (HSV3 or varicella zoster), this beast creates a neurological condition that goes away in young people over the course of two weeks, while it becomes a chronic condition in older adults. Old people and those with compromised immune systems often have to deal with it for life.

Although unlikely, is it possible for this chronic rash to be a reanimation of an unknown herpetic infection, one we don't know of yet? As new vaccines become available, so do new mutations. Rosea and roseola come to mind.

Chronic rashes may be promulgated this way, yet patients do better after an aggressive heavy metal detox. Infections and genetic predispositions seem to be just pieces of the puzzle. Foods, stress and toxins matter more.

Zinc Oxide -- Cheap and Effective

Zinc oxide, the white, thick cream commonly thought of as diaper rash cream or sunscreen, turns out, is antifungal, antiviral and antibacterial. The non-nano version in powder form may offer wonderful benefits when applied to mucosal membranes, while the thick cream version is great for all external skin conditions. Combine with Lysine and you may find additional relief.

Lysine can be taken internally, in a pill form. It can also be crushed and applied topically. Lysine is an amino acid that has been clinically proven to ameliorate herpetic infections.

Topical applications of crystalline lysine therapy have proven that the L-lysine-treated skin remains normal, "whereas untreated controls manifested clinical symptoms suggesting that an immunomodulatory effect of L-lysine is possible.[16]

Although sometime is being spent here on herpes viruses, the quickly growing chronic "yeast" infection is most likely, not a viral infection long term. Viral infections are easy to establish. In many of the cases I have dealt with, patients also feel that urine and bodily fluids reignite it. That would be the case if mercury, lead, aluminum, cadmium and other heavy metal toxins are being excreted through the urine and the bodily fluids in the area.

Detoxing the Kidneys and the Bladder

Heavy metal toxins accumulate in the kidneys. That is a well known fact, confirmed by researchers from Université de Nice-Sophia Antipolis, Nice, France, who also assert that "these non-essential elements are toxic at very low doses and non-biodegradable with a very long biological half-life."

Heavy metals present a serious health hazard and the kidneys are the first major organs that suffer because of their ability to accumulate and reabsorb metals.

How do we detox the kidneys and the bladder?

Through the centuries, the common method of detox has been through clay, charcoal, cilantro, nettle, baking soda, and goldenrod (solidago).

A very important element, not to be omitted, is Chlorella -- the antiviral, detoxing, chelating, glutathione supporting, high in amino acids and gut repairing supper-substance known to man.

Cilantro has its own chelation benefits as a highly effective metal toxin binding agent, an anti-inflammatory and antibacterial agent that prevents gas, bloating and nausea. It is also an expectorant high in iron and magnesium that supports liver health.

Unfortunately, one or two pills a day will not make a difference. A fully aggressive, physician supervised protocol must be implemented.[17]

Detox Protocol

To recap, there are a number of ways for one to detox heavy metals, but first a proper diagnosis is needed. Toxicities are associated with the following symptoms:

- Brain Fog
- Digestive irregularities (bloating, constipation, diarrhea)
- Memory loss
- Chronic sore throat
- Systemic inflammation
- Hair loss
- Rashes, often where bodily fluids are present
- Chronic yeast infections
- Anorexia
- Burning or clogged nasal passages
- Breathing problems

- Loss of balance, tremmors and /or dizziness
- Constant low grade depression (loss of zest for life)
- Anxiety and/or insomnia
- Autoimmune conditions, including Lyme Disease
- Eye irritation
- Chronic fatigue
- Headaches
- High blood pressure, and more

WHEN TO DETOX: If you have an *established* heavy metal toxicity, you must detox. There are a number of medications available with prescription. There are also powerful plants, EDTA, DMSA, melatonin creams and suppositories, vitamin C drops, glutathione sprays, taurine, NAC and vitamin C drops that can help you with the detoxification process. *Please get properly diagnosed. There are many conditions that share the above symptoms.*

Foods that bond and expel heavy metals include:

BREAKFAST: oatmeal, pears, grapes, plums, papayas, green apples, citrus fruit, pomegranates.

LUNCH AND DINNER: brown rice, whole grains, quinoa, peas, beans (all kinds), chickpeas, onions, garlic, bok choy, cabbage, broccoli, cauliflower, Brussel sprouts, carrots, spinach, cilantro, turmeric, parsley, dill, basil, thyme, ginger.

HERBS: spirulina, chlorella, burdock root, zeolite, shilajit, milk thistle, dandelion, barley grass, Atlantic dulse, nettle, charcoal, clay, cilantro, turmeric.

Supplements must be adjusted based on your individual test results.

INSTRUCTIONS:

1. Eat only these foods for a week. Take stock and be in constant contact with your doctor.
2. Soak feet in ionic foot spa for 20 minutes every night.
3. If no contraindications are present, use a dry heat sauna for 30 minutes each day (or wrap yourself in 3 blankets while soaking feet to induce sweat before rinsing the entire body off).
4. Sleep on a grounding pillow.

5. Drink unsweetened dandelion tea made with clean, metal-free water throughout the day.
6. Turn off your WiFi router while you sleep. If you have a Smart Meter, turn off the electricity to the room where you sleep altogether. Do not keep wireless (not just cell) phones around. In fact, go back to a corded phone.
7. Keep all wireless devices turned off where you sleep.
8. Take a multivitamin (that includes B12, full spectrum of minerals, and Omega-3) daily.

There are many, many methods of cleansing that could be added to the list, but this is a good place to start. In some cases, the symptoms may get worse before they get better. That is a known, common occurrence known as a Herxheimer reaction.

The most important factors are time, persistence and physician support. Heavy metals are tough to detox and re-contamination often continues to be a problem. Please don't give up.

To your health!

Disclaimer: Not intended to treat, prevent or diagnose any condition. Consult your physician prior to starting any new nutritional or supplement regimen. There are many contraindications that need to be considered.

References

1. ABDA Authors (2018) Basics of Behcet's Disease. Retrieved from http://www.behcets.com/site/c.8oIJJRPsGcISF/b.9196317/k.904C/Behcets_Disease.htm

2. WebMD authors (2005-2019) Why Do I Have a Rash Near My Vagina? Retrieved from https://www.webmd.com/sexual-conditions/rash-near-vagina#1

3. Harris, Victoria, Fischer, Gayle (2017) Sudden Onset of Painful Genital Ulcers

Retrieved from https://medicinetoday.com.au/dermatology-quiz/sudden-onset-painful-genital-ulcers

4.Care Down There, Aphthous Ulcers. Retrieved from http://www.caredownthere.com.au/_pages/advice_ulcers.html

5.Justin J. Finch, MD[1]; Jenna Wald, MD[2]; Katalin Ferenczi, MD (November 2014) Disseminated Lyme Disease Presenting With Nonsexual Acute Genital Ulcers
Retrieved from https://jamanetwork.com/journals/jamadermatology/fullarticle/1899258

6. Radcliff, Shawn (January 4, 2018) Lyme Disease Able to Survive 28-Day Antibiotic Treatment. Retrieved from https://www.healthline.com/health-news/lyme-disease-able-to-survive-antibiotic-treatment

7. Mercola (February 5. 2012) Why is Lyme Disease Not JUST a Tick-Borne Disease Any

More? Retrieved from https://articles.mercola.com/sites/articles/archive/2012/02/05/dr-dietrich-klinghardt-on-lyme-disease.aspx

8. Hardell and Carlberg (2017), Peleg et al., 2018, Miller et al 2018. Retrieved from https://www.hindawi.com/journals/bmri/2017/9218486/ .

9. EMF Solutions (July 3, 2017) Mold Produces 600 Times More Bio-Toxins with EMF. Retrieved from https://emfsol.com/mold-produces-600-times-more-bio-toxins-with-emf/

10. Brewer JH1, Thrasher JD, Straus DC, Madison RA, Hooper D. (April 11, 2013) Detection of Mycotoxins in Patients with Chronic Fatigue Syndrome. Retrieved from https://www.ncbi.nlm.nih.gov/pubmed/23580077

11. Liew WP1, Mohd-Redzwan S1 (February 26, 2018) Mycotoxin: Its Impact on Gut Health and Microbiota. Retrieved from https://www.ncbi.nlm.nih.gov/pubmed/29535978

12. Ross, Marty MD (2019) Control Cytokines: A Guide to Fix Lyme Symptoms & The Immune System. Retrieved from https://www.treatlyme.net/guide/cytokines

13. Ross, Marty MD (2019) Mold and Lyme Toxin Illness. Retrieved from https://www.treatlyme.net/guide/mold-toxin-illness-lyme-toxin

14. Anna Dittfeld, Katarzyna Gwizdek, Marek Michalski, and Romuald Wojnicz (October 25, 2016) A Possible Link Between the Epstein-Barr Virus Infection and Autoimmune Thyroid Disorders. Retrieved from https://www.ncbi.nlm.nih.gov/pmc/articles/PMC5099387/

15. Tzhaki, Ruth F. (October 19, 2018) Corroboration of a Major Role for Herpes Simplex Virus Type 1 in Alzheimer's Disease. Retrieved from https://www.ncbi.nlm.nih.gov/pmc/articles/PMC6202583/

16. Ayala E, Krikorian D. (May 28, 1989) Effect of L-lysine Monohydrochloride on Cutaneous Herpes Simplex Virus in the Guinea Pig. Retrieved from https://www.ncbi.nlm.nih.gov/pubmed/2542441

17. Barbier O, Jacquillet G, Tauc M, Cougnon M, Poujeol P.(February 17, 2005) Effect of Heavy Metals on, and Handling by, the Kidney. Retrieved from https://www.ncbi.nlm.nih.gov/pubmed/15722646